Blood, Sweat, and Prayers:

The Spirit, Soul, and Body Connection to Weight Loss

Blood, Sweat, and Prayers:

The Spirit, Soul, and Body Connection to Weight Loss

Keri Watkins Webb

Published by Keri Watkins Webb 9/12/2017
Empowered Living
www.empoweredlivingnyc.com

ISBN-13: 978-1975657147
ISBN-10: 1975657144

Disclaimer:

The health information presented in this book is based on training, personal experience, and research. The author of this book does not dispense medical advice or prescribe the use or the discontinuance of any medications as a form of treatment without the advice of an attending physician, either directly or indirectly. All of the recommendations and procedures herein contained are made without guarantee on the part of the author or the publisher, their agents, or employees. The author and publisher disclaim all liability in connection with the use of information presented herein.

Because of the dynamic nature of the Internet, any web addresses or links contained in this book may have changed since publication and may no longer be valid.

I dedicate this book to both of my fathers – who art in Heaven.

Contents

Acknowledgements

To My Mother: Thank you for bringing me into this world and always putting my needs above your own. You have always been my biggest cheerleader!

To My Father: Thank you for teaching me to serve.

To Kara and Emmanuel: Thank you for always supporting me and loving me unconditionally.

To Elysia and Amadia: Thank you for all you are becoming.

To Kelly, Nika, Cynthia, Rosalyn, Tanine, Tracey, Judi, and Maria: Thank you for your continued love, encouragement, wisdom, and support.

To Troy, Daniel, Leroy, Steve and Dave: Thank you for always believing in me and having my back. You are the big brothers I never had.

To Matt: Thank you for your honesty and for always encouraging me to seek deeper depths and higher heights.

To Ray: We have run the gamut of experiences—from erecting bars on my basement window to sitting in meetings with city councilmen. Through it all you have helped me to live fuller, laugh louder, and look deeper. Thank you for always protecting me. You are my "ride or die" forever friend.

To Kevin and Jordan: Although I didn't give you the gift of life, your lives have been a tremendous gift to me. Thank you for making "motherhood" easy.

To My Extended Family: Thank you to all of my aunts, uncles, and cousins (too many to name) for guiding me and shaping me throughout my journey.

To My Husband: Thank you for always seeing the best in me and accepting me just as I am.

To God: Thank you for saving me and helping me to move beyond my self-imposed boundaries.

Author's Note

By nature I am impatient. I could not wait to graduate high school. I could not wait to get my driver's license. I could not wait to turn 21. I could not wait to live independently. I could not wait to become a teacher. But, by far, my biggest challenge was that I could not wait to lose weight.

My impatience prompted me to try every diet fad and exercise plan known to man. As a result, I embarked upon the emotional and physical roller-coaster of yo-yo dieting. But, when I surrendered my life to God and developed a close, personal relationship with Him, I learned patience, and about the wisdom of waiting.

In addition to waiting, I also began watching. In Luke 21:36, Jesus cautions us to "watch and pray always." Because God's way requires constant vigilance, I learned to keep my guard up at all times, lest I succumb to the same old dieting pitfalls of the past. My "antenna" also remained up, in order to ensure that what I was hearing was true. My primary questions: *What were the proper foods to eat? What type of exercise plan would be most beneficial? Which health sources were the most reliable? From whom should I seek counsel?*

When my vision became focused, my hearing became clear, and my palate became discriminatory, I was able to achieve my weight loss goals. I adopted a healthy lifestyle and lost 48 pounds to boot! While many may contend that I was successful because I "watched my weight," I maintain that successful weight loss only occurs when one waits, watches, and prays. And, so, l encourage you to become a "wait watcher", and discover how to permanently eliminate dieting from your life.

Introduction

The Spirit, Soul, Body Connection

3 John 2 states: *"Beloved, above all I wish that you prosper and be in good health even as your soul prospers."* This scripture reveals God's desire for his children to thrive in spirit, soul, and body. Just as God cautions us to consistently safeguard the gateways to our heart (Proverbs 4:23), in order to ensure spiritual prosperity, we are also urged to protect these entry ways to ensure maximum health and wellness. This correlation is clearly outlined in the charts below:

Literal Parallels

Spiritual Gateways to the Heart	Physical Gateways to the Body
Mouth- used to edify, praise, pray	Mouth – used to consume proper foods
Ears – used to receive positive messages	Ears – used to listen to recommendations of health care providers, personal trainers and other professionals
Eyes – used to read truth, watch positive images	Eyes – used to look at food as a source of nourishment and strength.

Symbolic Parallels

Spiritual Gateways to the Heart	Physical Gateways to the Body
Mouth- represents a fountain of blessings or a vessel of truth	Mouth – represents an entrance to the temple of God
Ears – represent receipt of wisdom	Ears –represent the need to listen to your body
Eyes – represent search for truth	Eyes – represent a ncw perception/perspective on food and health

This chart outlines a simple yet practical, three-tiered approach to successful weight loss:

1. The Eyes – must gain a new perspective
2. The Mouth – must consume proper foods, and
3. The Ears--must receive wisdom.

These three tenets can also be described as the *spirit*, *soul* and *body* connection to weight loss. In other words, in order to lose weight and keep it off, all three facets of man's being must be in alignment: the soul must be renewed, the body must be disciplined and the spirit must be revealed.

Part One: Spirit

Chapter 1

Uncovering the Holy Spirit

"Don't you know that you yourselves are God's temple and that God's spirit lives in you?"

–1 Corinthians 3:16-17

Recently, I attended an empowerment workshop. There I was introduced to the theoretical concept, "The Pie of Knowledge." This ideology is rooted in the notion that a person's knowledge base is divided into three distinct areas: That which we know, that which we don't know, and that which we are totally unaware of. The latter section, which is the largest division, represents all things unseen and all things yet to be revealed. While the developers of this theory claim that this area is governed by our subconscious, I believe that it is led by the Holy Spirit.

When applying this theoretical framework to my life, I discovered that for most of my life, my knowledge base was limited to the first two regions of this "Pie." Endowed with a good mind and a strong body, I had learned to think for myself, to take initiative, and to rely on my own abilities. Many times I failed, falling short of my own expectations. My response was always the same: Set your will, study more, work harder, and do better next time. When my efforts proved to be fruitful, I credited luck and hard work for my success.

The church I attended somehow failed to impart (to me) the concept of a personal relationship with God. Although I was involved in many activities, church was nothing more than a chore which I performed on Sundays. I recited prayers that I learned by rote and kneeled and bowed at the appropriate times. Religiously, every Tuesday, I recited nine Hail Mary's before noon in hopes of receiving a special blessing. Needless to say, when my expectations were not met, I was extremely disappointed. But nevertheless, I continued with this ritual believing that if I prayed harder I would garner more positive results.

After several disappointing Tuesdays, I concluded that religion had nothing to offer me. By this point, my relationship with God was reduced to an occasional prayer at mealtime and a plea for help in moment of despair. My actions and their consequences were direct reflections of my emotions. I would feel—then act—then think. This cyclic pattern of self-destructions plagued my adolescence and spilled over into my adulthood. It resulted in low self-esteem, shame, worry, doubt, guilt, deception, and physical illness.

Although I looked happy on the outside, I was miserable on the inside. I devoted all of my energy to developing my career, pursuing community activities, and keeping up with my social calendar. I kept my mind occupied night and day so that I did not have to deal with my empty reality.

Then one day when I was left alone to think about my situation, I began to sob uncontrollably. I lay in bed and cried out to God: "Please, help me!" Suddenly the whole atmosphere in my room changed. There was a Presence there, powerful, comforting, and peaceful. Then as mysteriously as it entered, it left. Although my room was normal again, something inside of me was different.

Shortly thereafter, a series of events occurred: a co-worker invited me to read the Bible with her during her lunch hour; a friend sent me a subscription to a Christian magazine; another friend invited me to go to church with her. Although these gestures had been extended to me before, I had always rejected them. This time, I said, "yes." This marked the beginning of my walk with God.

In July of 1996, I started going to church on a regular basis. This church, although a large departure from what I remembered church as being, felt like home. While the teachings from the sermons helped to enhance my perspective, the gospel music stirred my soul. I looked forward to the fellowship and traveled over 30 miles, each week, rain or shine, to partake in it. No longer a chore, church had become a vital and integral part of life, which helped to solidify my relationship with God. In January of the following year, I publicly signified this relationship, through the sacrament of Baptism.

A few months later, God took me one step farther. He made it clear that I had to surrender myself entirely to Him. This was a struggle. My will was well-developed and strong. Finally, I acknowledged, that by doing things my way I had not achieved tremendous success. Although I had earned two graduate degrees and had excellent career prospects, my social life was problematic. I needed inner peace and fulfillment. It seemed there was no alternative but to surrender.

Although I knew that this was the right thing to do, it was a difficult process. But God, in His infinite wisdom, helped me to surrender one aspect of my life at a time. First, He helped me to surrender my body. I understood that the time had come to modify my eating habits and adopt an exercise regimen. For the first time in my life, I began to view my body as a temple and began to treat it as such. I then made the connection that my body was the vehicle through which I could physically manifest God's will; thus, in order to do His will, my body had to be strong. With this new insight, surrendering my body became easy, and this newly acquired discipline soon trickled over into my spiritual life.

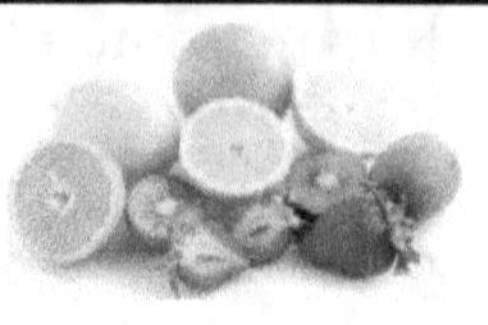

View your body as a temple and begin to treat it as such. Your body is the vehicle through which you can physically manifest God's will; thus, in order to do His will, your body must be strong. When you understand this, surrendering your body will become easy.

Realizing that my ears, eyes, and mouth were the gateways to my heart, I began to listen, watch, and speak God's Word. I began watching Christian programming on television; I attended spiritual retreats; I listened to teaching tapes; and I began witnessing for God. I soon developed the ability to discern between positive and negative habits and fruitful and destructive relationships. I took inventory of my life and discarded all things that were not in agreement with God's will. I had fallen in love with God and nothing satisfied me except His word.

The new life I had acquired astonished me. Doubts and fears dissipated and suddenly I was able to make every change God had asked in absolute assurance that He would stand behind me. During my years alone I had become a very independent person. Now, I had learned a new dependence on the Holy Spirit. I knew I could not obey the Lord unless I heard His voice; a holy awe and fear kept me seeking Him lest I should fail for lack of attentiveness.

When I allowed God to increase in my life, everything else began to decrease—my ego, my pride, my worries, my fears, and yes, even my dress size! As my relationship with Him deepened, and as I learned to know His voice more clearly, God led me to adopt a proper eating regimen, to study nutrition, open a women's fitness center, teach a health course, and ultimately write this book!

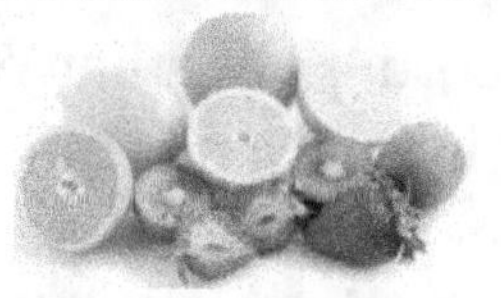

If you want to improve your physical health, I recommend that you begin by improving your spiritual health. To sum it all up, if you want to lose weight, stop focusing your attention on your body, and shift your attention toward developing a relationship with the Creator who gave it to you.

So, if you want to improve your physical health, I recommend that you begin by improving your spiritual health. I offer my story as one example of how God got my attention, loved me, and then drew me into a close, personal relationship. Although your experience will be different from mine, I think it will benefit you to begin to piece together your own account of getting to know God.

To sum it all up, if you want to lose weight, stop focusing your attention on your body, and shift your attention toward developing a relationship with the Creator who gave it to you. Begin by reviewing your lifeline. Meditate on the different shifts in your life and ask yourself why things happened as they did, why certain people came into your life, and where God might have been in those instances. The details of how God comes to us are not important—what matters is that we are open enough to receive Him.

Prayer:

Lord, I pray that You would order my steps. Lead me in Your light, teach me Your way, so that I will walk in Your truth. Help me to have a deeper walk with You and an ever-progressing hunger for Your Word. I pray this prayer In Jesus' precious name. Amen.

Chapter 2

Making the Connection: Why Diets Fail

"I am a part of a royal priesthood and a nation that belongs to God; therefore, what the world says about me is not God's opinion of who I am."

−1 Peter 2:9

After dieting for many years and never experiencing long-term success, I came to the conclusion that most diets fail because they are based on physical and food-oriented methods. Although this approach to weight loss seems "logical", the truth is, we must see ourselves as more than physical beings.

It has been said that we are *"spirit beings having a human experience."* In other words, we are spirits who have minds and occupy bodies. Yes, the three facets of ourselves are quite intimately related. It is not until we align our mind and spirit with our body's weight loss goals that we will achieve permanent results.

In recent years, Western science has become increasingly more aware that its approach to health care is fundamentally flawed. At the same time, we have discovered what Eastern medicine has known for centuries: Our health can only be optimized when the three aspects of self are in balance. An approach to health and healing that involves all three aspects of self (spirit, soul, and body) is called holistic. Etymology teaches us that the word holistic stems from the same root word as whole, hale and holy. So, in order to succeed at achieving optimal health and wholeness, we need to work with **all** of who we are. And to do that, we need to alter our backward priorities.

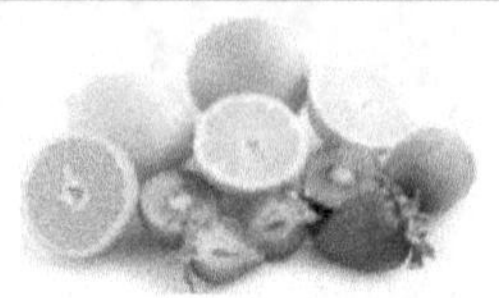

Our health can only be optimized when the three aspects of self are in balance. An approach to health and healing that involves all three aspects of self (spirit, soul, and body) is called holistic.

If you were reared in Western culture, you probably have some priorities that are not beneficial to your overall health and wellness. Society teaches us to become so focused on the trappings of the material world that we can barely acknowledge the non-physical one, let alone look to it for healing.

2 Timothy 4:3-4 says, *"For the time will come when men will not put up with sound doctrine. Instead, to suit their own desires, they will gather around them a great number of teachers to say what their itching ears want to hear. They will turn their ears away from the truth and turn aside to myths."*

Weight-loss campaigns boast expressions like, "Lose 10 pounds in 10 days." Or, "wear a magic girdle that will enable you to lose weight while you are sleeping." Although these diet fads are myths, they embody concepts we want to hear. And, because we want to hear them, we regard them as truth. In doing so, however, we set ourselves up for the only outcome we can expect if we base our actions on lies: failure.

Most of us have become overly concerned with reaching "a place called there"-- the place that signifies that we have "arrived" in life. This concept speaks to our preoccupation with attaining "worldly" status and attaining material possessions. It is the illusory nature of this physical world—a belief that what you can see is much more meaningful and much more powerful than that which you cannot see.

Quantum Theory, a branch of the physical science, has discovered that, no matter how closely we look, we never really find anything "solid." So, if we buy into the illusion--that what we can see is what's "real"—we will never discover that what we can't see--the entire spiritual realm--is even more real.

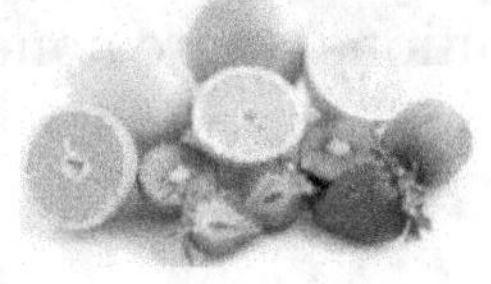

Our inaccurate perceptions have resulted in inaccurate priorities. Our inaccurate priorities have compelled us to look to the wrong sources for solutions. And the result of looking in the wrong place for solutions, is that we end up with excess weight that we can't get rid of, health problems that we shouldn't have, and a great deal of stress that could have been avoided.

It all boils down to a problem in perception. We have learned to believe that the physical world is more real than the spiritual one. And, indeed, to our earthly eyes, it "looks" more real. But, our blindness to other realms of reality, that are actually more important, is what's keeping us stuck at a weight we don't like.

To sum it all up, our inaccurate perceptions have resulted in inaccurate priorities. Our inaccurate priorities have compelled us to look to the wrong sources for solutions. And the result of looking in the wrong place for solutions, is that we end up with excess weight that we can't get rid of, health problems that we shouldn't have, and a great deal of stress that could have been avoided.

In order to put an end to this cyclical pattern of self-destruction, we have to adopt a major shift in perception. We must understand that what we cannot see is actually more powerful and more influential in our lives than what we can see. Unless we grasp this essential concept, we will always be seeking solutions where none exist.

Prayer:

Lord, grant me wisdom in every decision I make. Help me to seek Your ways and seek to know the truth. Give me discernment to make decisions based on Your revelation and not the foolishness of this world. Help me to keep my eyes focused on You so that my perception and priorities are clear. In Jesus' name, I pray. Amen.

Chapter 3

Increasing Your Spiritual Health

*"The Spirit gives life; the flesh counts for
nothing. The words I have spoken to you are
spirit and they are life."*

–John 6:63

Faith is a gift from God. However, we often become so consumed with the busyness of life that we neglect our spiritual growth. We yearn to know God on a deeper level but, our lifestyle choices sometimes make this virtually impossible. We become distracted by anything and everything: work, media, chores, parenting, socializing, hobbies, etc. If we want to develop a meaningful relationship with God, we have to be intentional. It's just like developing a relationship with a friend, spouse, or co-worker. It takes time and effort. Proverbs 13:4 says, *"The sluggard craves and gets nothing, but the desires of the diligent are fully satisfied."* Your relationship with God cannot be a preference—it must be a conviction. It has to be as important as going to work, raising your children, or socializing with friends.

Romans 8:6 says, "For to be carnally minded is death; but to be spiritually minded is life and peace." The word "carnal" in this scripture does not necessarily mean sinful. It means physical – concerned with the flesh and the human frailties of man (see James Strong's, The Exhaustive Concordance of the Bible [Nashville: Abingdon, 1890], Greek Dictionary of the New Testament, #4561). This scripture shows us, if we are carnally minded, we will die. But, if we are spiritually minded, we will have life and peace. Take a moment to reflect on your life. Are you experiencing life and peace? Spiritual-mindedness produces peace the same way that planting tomato seeds produces tomatoes. You don't plant tomato seeds and get corn. You reap what you sow. What is true in agriculture is true in life. Whatever you are experiencing or harvesting in your life is a direct reflection of what you've been focusing on.

Isaiah 26:3 says, "Thou wilt keep him in perfect peace, whose mind is stayed on thee: because he trusteth in thee." This scripture reveals that our sense of peace is not determined by our outward circumstances but, rather, by our inward thoughts. If we think about the negative things of this world, we will become depressed because the realities of this world can be grim. But, if we think about the positive things of God, we will have perfect peace.

The Bible says that we are not to be conformed to this world but rather we are to be transformed by renewing our mind (Proverbs 23:7). The Bible helps us to renew our minds which will change the way we think. In other words: read the Bible and it will change how you think and that, in turn, will change you.

The Bible is not merely for reading, however, it should be studied so that it can be applied. Otherwise, it is like swallowing food without chewing and then regurgitating it—no nutritional value is gained from it. Meditating on the Word daily draws us closer to God and helps us to see life from His perspective—the right perspective.

However, I caution you—God's perspective is often in direct opposition to the natural way of thinking. For example, the Bible tells us to love our enemies and forgive those who have hurt us. The Bible tells us that we are fundamentally sinful and that our hearts are deceitful. The Bible warns us not to become too proud or haughty and reminds us to serve others with humility.

These are different ideas. The Bible is full of different ideas. But as you read and embrace these concepts, they will change the way you think and how you respond to life's circumstances. But, you cannot read the Bible periodically and expect these results. In order to transform your mind, yourself, and your life, you need to immerse yourself in Bible studies.

The following is a list of 10 habits that will help you to deepen your relationship with God through the study of His Word:

1. **Make Bible Study a Priority.** Read the Bible daily so that God's Word will become inscribed in your heart. (*As a man thinketh in his heart, so is he--* Proverbs 23:7).

2. **Pray Before and After Bible Study.** Ask God to open up your mind and heart to what He wants to reveal to you. This simple step can help make scripture come "alive" and help you to interpret text.

3. **Avoid Bible Study Schedules.** Specific guides and plans may require you to cover large amounts of

scripture in one sitting. Study at your own pace so that you can fully digest what you are reading.

4. **Use Dictionaries, Commentaries and Concordances to Help You Comprehend the Bible.** It is difficult to learn the Bible without proper guidance. Even Biblical scholars rely on various resources in order to gain understanding.

5. **Arrange to Have Some Quiet Time Every Day.** Fifteen uninterrupted minutes is better than an hour of distracted study. Dedicate a specific place and time for your Bible study. It is best to develop a daily routine or schedule for this practice.

6. **Don't Despair If You Do Not Understand Everything.** Even Bible scholars debate about certain verses. Study what you can and make a note of those concepts you don't understand immediately. Hopefully, you will understand them at some point in the future.

7. **If You Miss a Day or Two of Bible Study, Don't Stop.** Don't waste any more time feeling guilty about missed study. Get back to the Bible as soon as possible.

8. **Put What You Learn into Practice.** As you understand how to apply Biblical principles, your study will be more compelling.

9. **Use Different Techniques to Enhance Your Study.** Methods like journaling, praying God's word and establishing a study group will help to enrich your study.

10. **Share What You Learn with Others.** Share Biblical truths with friends, family, and other people that are put in your path. The world is hungry for God's Word.

It is important to remember that these habits are not ends in themselves but a means to the end of knowing God more deeply. Evangelist Joseph Prince illustrates this point best, during one of his teachings: "Let's look at the word "habit." If you remove the "h" you still have "a bit." If you remove the "a" you still have "bit." If you remove the "b" you still have "it." When you remove "i" all that's left is "t" or the Cross. In other words, when you remove yourself or "I" and look to the Cross, the Bible study process becomes less about your performance and more about your interdependence on God."

Prayer:

Lord, ignite my spiritual life so that I may know you better. Help me to remain committed to you and make You a priority in my life. Empower me to stay away from anything or anybody who might take your place in my heart. Open my eyes and ears to receive wisdom and help me to understand your Word and how it applies to my life. I pray this prayer, in Jesus' name. Amen.

Chapter 4

Fear vs. Faith

"Do not be afraid or discouraged because of this vast army. For the battle is not yours, but God's."

–2 Chronicles 20:15

In 2005, I took a great leap of faith—I bought a women's fitness franchise. This was the biggest decision I had ever made. While contemplating the pros and the cons of this new venture, I entertained all of the "what if" scenarios in my head. What if I fail? What if I lose my money? What if I can't juggle all of my responsibilities? The list was endless. Then one day, after listening to the negative script I repeatedly rehearsed, my friend said, "Do it afraid. What's the worst thing that can happen?" Those two statements, as simple as they may seem, revolutionized my thought pattern; I began to view all of the worst case scenarios much differently. I decided that if I failed, I would learn from my mistakes and start again; if I lost money, I would use my investments to cover my debts; if I wasn't able to handle my responsibilities, I would eliminate some of my duties or seek help. But, most importantly, I began to ask myself, what would happen if I allow fear to rob me of my dreams? The answer: I would live to regret it.

Motivational speaker, Tony Robbins says the only way you can live fearlessly is to die. If this is true, we are never totally liberated from fear during our lifetime. And although faith in God doesn't necessarily guarantee freedom from fear, it does empower us to defuse fear's control over us and frees us to accomplish everything God desires for us to do and achieve.

If you think about the faithful figures of the Bible you will see that faith empowered them to do what God had called them to do. Here's what the Word says about them: "By faith Noah ... By faith Abraham ... By faith Isaac ... By faith Jacob ... By faith Joseph ... By faith Moses ... By faith the people passed through the Red Sea ... By faith the walls of Jericho fell down... By faith Gideon, Barak, Samson, Jephthah, David, and Samuel all conquered kingdoms, administered justice, and gained what was promised.

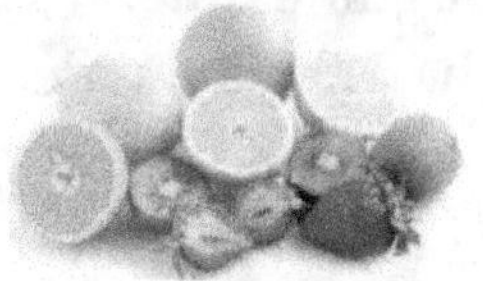

What false evidence do you use to justify your internal dialogue concerning your health? What are you afraid of when it comes to changing your health habits? Are you afraid that you will fail? Are you afraid to get out of your comfort zone? Maybe you're afraid that you won't be able to socialize anymore. Maybe you think it will be too hard. Whatever your fear is, if you want to adopt a healthier lifestyle, you must face it.

Although all of us are not called to do great things for God, all of us are called to bring glory to God through our actions. To achieve this we need faith. And just like change is a choice, faith is a choice. It is a choice to put our trust in God (despite our fears) and to do what David chose to do. He prayed to God, "When I am afraid, I will trust in you..."

When our journey is over, may it also be said of you and me, "By faith ______________________________________ (put your name in the blank space) overcame his/her challenges and achieved his/her goals.

Philippians 4:13 says, "I can do all things through Christ who strengthens me." Trusting in God's wisdom strengthens your faith. When you decide to step out in faith, you learn that God is with you wherever you go and that God is more powerful than your fear. So, next time you are urged to do something and you decide to take a leap of faith, focus on the Cross. When you relinquish control and submit yourself to God, you will actually find freedom.

It has been said that the acronym for the word FEAR is: *False Evidence Appearing Real.* This means that the only thing stopping you from accomplishing your goals is the false evidence or the fabricated story you continually tell yourself. What false evidence do you use to justify your internal dialogue? What are you afraid of when it comes to changing your health habits? Are you afraid that you will fail? Are you afraid to get out of your comfort zone? Maybe you're afraid that you won't be able to socialize anymore. Maybe you think it will be too hard. Whatever your fear is, if you want to adopt a healthier lifestyle, you must face it. Evangelist Paula White says that you can't conquer what you don't confront and you can't confront that which you don't identify.

Spend some time reflecting on this chapter.

What fears do you need to identify and overcome?

____

____

____

Prayer:

Lord, I pray that fear will not rule over me. Instead, may Your Word penetrate every fiber of my being and convince me that Your love for me is far greater than anything I face. I pray this prayer in Jesus' precious name. Amen.

Part Two: Soul
The Mind, Will, and Emotions

Chapter 1

Rewriting Your Script

"Let no foul or polluting language, nor evil word nor unwholesome or worthless talk [ever] come out of your mouth but only [speech] as is good and beneficial to the spiritual progress of others, as is fitting to the need and the occasion, that it may be a blessing and give grace to those who hear it."

–Ephesians 4:29

Whether we tweet, text, instant message or e-mail, we are all published authors. We express our opinions about sports teams, current events, politics, music, religion, and even injustices that we may encounter on a daily basis. Sometimes we report our "status" or share significant events in our lives. Other times we use social media to network, advertise, and market ourselves and our personal pursuits. Whatever the purpose, most of us feel the need to express our viewpoint. Unfortunately, however, our comments are rarely, if ever, edited. Typically, we shoot from the hip without giving our sentiments much thought.

Reverend Dale Bronner uses the acronym "THINK" to describe the way we should express ourselves. He says our words should always be True, Helpful, Insightful, Necessary, and Kind. We should use our words to uplift and edify, never to tear down or destroy. But, how often do we use our words to criticize and condemn? We are almost always aware of the impact of our words when we direct them towards others, but we are rarely aware of the ramifications of our words when directed at ourselves.

During my 20's and 30's I was very hard on myself, and often put myself down. While I would never dream of verbally abusing or even harshly criticizing others, I thought it was perfectly acceptable to treat myself in this manner. So, while other people thought well of me and seemed to hold me in high regard, I couldn't understand why I felt unhappy most of the time and suffered from low self-esteem. It wasn't until I recognized that my identity was wrapped in Christ that I began to see myself the way that He sees me – as a woman of true value and worth. And so, I searched the scriptures to find out everything that God said about me and began to speak about myself accordingly. I made a list of these Biblical affirmations and recited them daily until they were committed to memory. Whenever I would feel discouraged, I would revisit the list to remind myself of the thoughts I should be thinking.

In James 3:4-8, it is written: Even so, the tongue is a little member, and it can boast of great things. See how much wood or how great a forest a tiny spark can set ablaze...but the human tongue can be tamed by no man. It is a restless (undisciplined) evil, full of deadly poison.

As this passage states, no man can tame their own tongue—not by themselves, anyway. That's why we need the help of God. Without God, we cannot change anything. But, when we agree with Him, all things are possible. (Matthew 17:20). Simply, take the Word of God and start to speak it over your life. Instead of saying, "I will never lose weight," "Nobody will want me," or "I give up", begin saying, "I can do all things through Christ who strengthens me," "I am beautifully and wonderfully made," and "I am more than a conqueror."

Be selective in your speech for words are containers of power. The kind of power is contingent upon the kind of words you choose. You can curse your future by speaking negatively about it, or you can bless it by speaking positively about it. Negative self-talk will usually lead to anxiety and depression. This type of conversation is so powerful that it leads to self-fulfilling prophecies: You start believing your own propaganda and bring about what you say. Fortunately, the converse is also true. Positive self-talk will tend to achieve desirable outcomes and generate good feelings.

So, does it help to change what you say to yourself? It certainly does. Tell yourself often enough that you'll fail and you almost certainly will. Tell yourself often enough that you'll succeed and you will greatly improve your chances of fulfillment and satisfaction. In fact, Dr. Clifford N. Lazarus says that successful people:

- Don't focus on failures
- See mistakes as learning experiences for growth and understanding
- Don't indulge in self-recrimination

He further suggests, the difference between the foolish and the wise, is not that the wise do not make mistakes. Rather, it is that the wise learn from their mistakes instead of telling themselves they're stupid for making them.

The bottom line: "Say unto yourself what you would have others say unto you."

What self-defeating phrases do you say about yourself?

____

____

How can you re-write those phrases as positive statements?

____

____

Prayer:

Heavenly Father, your Word says that whatsoever I desire when I pray, I should believe and receive, in the name of Jesus. Therefore, I pray now, in Jesus' name, that I am set free from negative thoughts and disparaging speech. As I have adopted the mind of Christ, I reject, refuse, and bind negative thoughts and statements and will only receive and speak words of faith. Today, I begin to be what God says I am. I am a person of authority, power, dominion, grace and favor. Thank you for encouraging me and supporting me on this journey. Amen.

Chapter 2

Managing Your Emotions

*"Create in me a pure heart, O God, and renew a
steadfast spirit within me."*

–Psalm 51:10

"Right thinking" leads to "right actions," which leads to
"right feelings." This hierarchy is critical. If feelings are at the
front, they will drive you wherever they feel like going. You've
heard it said, "If it feels this good, it must be the right thing to
do." Although it sounds good, this type of thinking is
problematic; your emotions will lead you into all kinds of chaos
and confusion. "Right thinking" guides us in responding with
"right actions." And, although right feelings may not come
immediately, they will come eventually.

Right thinking is based on seeing each situation from
God's point of view. In 2 Corinthians 4:16, Paul states, "For
which cause we faint not; but though our outward man perish,
yet the inward man is renewed day by day." In this scripture,
Paul reveals that although life can be problematic he will not be
controlled or dominated by the trappings of the world. The
power of God that resides inside him is more powerful than any

problem he may encounter in the physical realm. The spiritual side of Paul is what is truly alive-- so that is the part that he chooses to focus on. It will not perish, but it will be renewed every day.

Like Paul, if we are to overcome the emotions that attack us each day, we must keep this distinction clearly in mind.

4 Steps to Transforming Unhealthy Emotions

STEP 1: IDENTIFY YOUR UNHEALTHY EMOTION

2 Corinthians 10:5 provides a framework for how we can renew our minds: "We take captive every thought to make it obedient". In order to identify the thoughts that need to be taken captive we must first identify the thoughts that do not line up with God's Truth. This is actually simple. When we look at unhealthy emotions like jealousy, anger, fear, low self-esteem, etc. we can be sure there is a thought behind that emotion.

Go back in time for just a moment. Imagine you are five years old and a total stranger pokes you in the stomach and says, "Look at that fat little belly." Would you get mad? Probably not. You may have even giggled at the comment. However, with the same scenario fifteen years later your emotion would be totally different. Why? Because at age five your thought was, "this person is being friendly." However, at age 20 you wouldn't consider that person or their comment "friendly." You would probably be insulted. The same remark to the same person yields totally different results based on time, experience, and perspective.

The reality is, only our thoughts can create our emotions. So if our emotions are unhealthy we can be sure we have a thought that has not been taken captive. The easiest way to realize a thought has not been taken captive is to write down our unhealthy emotion and then begin to search for the thought that created this emotion.

STEP #2: WRITE DOWN THE THOUGHT THAT CREATED YOUR EMOTION

Once the unhealthy emotion has been identified we need to ask ourselves what the thought was that created that emotion. This requires us to be very attentive to our thoughts and feelings. Typically these thoughts enter our minds very quickly, so we have to pay close attention to them when they occur. These thoughts do not come from deep within us but they come from outside of us; they come from the world. 1 John 4:4 states, He that is in me is greater than he that is in the world."

It is critical for us to understand that when thoughts feel as if they are coming from outside us (from the world), they are not coming from God. These thoughts are extremely harmful and damage our psyche.

While I used to believe that these damaging thoughts were simply thoughts that didn't serve me well, I now know that every thought that results in an unhealthy emotion is a lie! Galatians 5:22-23 lists the fruits of the Spirit as: love, joy, peace, patience, kindness, goodness, faithfulness, gentleness, and self-control. These feelings are produced as a result of the Holy Spirit residing within us. So, if you have a thought that creates peace, it's reasonable to believe that it is coming from the Holy Spirit, which dwells in you. On the other hand, if a thought creates negative emotions such as anger, envy, strife, pride, jealousy, greed, etc., you can be sure that the thought is not coming from the Holy Spirit, but from the world. And, because the Holy "Spirit is the truth" (1 John 5:6), we can conclude that thoughts that create unhealthy emotions are lies and they cannot originate from God.

Our minds are constantly being bombarded with negative thoughts and lies. For example, have you ever had an argument with someone and continually replayed the incident over and over in your mind, imagining what you might have said to get your point across? You want to stop thinking about the interaction but you simply can't get it out of your mind. An argument that may have lasted several moments, has now taken up residence in your mind for several hours. The negative energy that you have devoted to this thought pattern will result in destructive emotions.

The next time you exchange negative thoughts or think negatively about a person or situation, instead of meditating on these emotions, write these thoughts down on paper. By writing them down, you will begin to obtain control over those thoughts or lies instead of allowing them to control you.

STEP #3: WRITE DOWN THE REPLACEMENT THOUGHT (THE TRUTH)

Once you recognize that unhealthy emotions are merely lies, you must replace each lie with the truth. Replacing thoughts with truth is a key component of the sanctification process. In John 17:17, Jesus makes this point clear when He asks His Father to "Sanctify them by the Truth."

Sometimes replacing lies with truth can be as simple as writing down the opposite thought of the one identified as a lie. For example, you might write, "I can't lose weight," in response to your unhealthy emotion of strife. And as a replacement thought you may simply write, "I have the freedom and ability to accomplish anything I decide to do." Another simple thought you may write that fits this pattern and analogy is, "My mate should lose weight," in response to your unhealthy emotion of judgment. As a replacement thought you might write, "My mate has the freedom to change any behavior that he/she desires. I will support him/her in whatever change he/she decides to undertake." It is important to note that the latter thought is not only the truth, but it also has the power to drastically change judgment into acceptance, a characteristic that has a tremendous amount of power to influence.

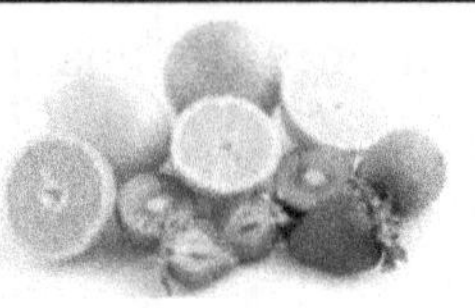

It is only by identifying and correcting the unhealthy, self-sabotaging thoughts and beliefs that are secretly creating unhealthy attitudes and behaviors, that one can heal their eating issues and restore their body Temple. This is precisely how the renewed mind will transform the physical body—by correcting the invisible source of eating problems once and for all—from the root!

By now, it may seem apparent that not all replacement thoughts are as simple as writing the opposite statement. In fact, at times it will be necessary for entire paradigms to shift in order to arrive at the truth. For instance, you may write, "I'm a loser," in response to your negative feeling of shame. Before writing down your replacement thought you may need to ask yourself a few questions: "How exactly do I define a loser?" If your response is, "a loser is a person that people don't like," then you have made great progress. The revelation that, "no one is liked by everyone" may soon become evident when you write your answer, and accordingly, you may realize that either everyone is a loser or your definition must somehow be skewed. In fact, as you continue to try and define "loser" you will continually become challenged. It is at this point, that a shift in thinking can occur – a shift from the Spirit. This is the defining moment when we open up to the Spirit and recognize that when we believe in God and invite Him into our lives, we actually become righteous. This point is specifically illustrated in Romans 4:24, where it is written, "but also for us, to whom God will credit righteousness—for us who believe in Him who raised Jesus our Lord from the dead." Therefore, if I am a believer it is impossible for me to be a loser, in fact, I am righteous...and if I'm righteous what makes me think I'm not good enough for myself? And is it reasonable to think that my opinion is more important than God's opinion of me? The answer is NO! Now you can document the truth. Your replacement thought may be, "As a believer in God I *become* the righteousness of God. And, if I am a righteous person, I cannot be a loser." Once again, the replacement thought is true and has the power of God to change self-contempt to love.

STEP #4: CONTINUALLY RE-READ THE REPLACEMENT THOUGHT (The Truth)

It is extremely important to recognize that replacing lies with truth is revelation **not** renewal. According to Holman's Bible Dictionary, revelation is "the content and process of God's making Himself known to people. All knowledge of God comes by way of revelation." Replacing lies with truth is procuring the knowledge of God because only truth can come from God. When truth is revealed, the opportunity for renewal begins. "Anakainosis" is the Greek word for renewing. It is important to note that "ana" as a prefix means repetition, intensity, and reversal (Strong's Hebrew & Greek Dictionary). It is this intense repetition of truth that results in the renewing of the mind.

It is only by identifying and correcting the unhealthy,

self-sabotaging thoughts and beliefs that are secretly creating unhealthy attitudes and behaviors, that one can heal their eating issues and restore their body Temple. This is precisely how the renewed mind will transform the physical body—by correcting the invisible source of eating problems once and for all—from the root!

Write down one unhealthy emotion (lie) you have told yourself.

____

Write down the replacement statement (truth).

____

Prayer:

Father God, thank you for loving me and accepting me for who I am. Whenever I allow the cares of this world to overshadow your love, grace, and acceptance, give me eyes to see and ears to hear the truth of Your Word. Guard my heart so that it remains open and receptive to the promptings of the Holy Spirit. And help me to remember that Your opinion is the only opinion that matters. May your thoughts be my thoughts and may I put the negative words of others where they belong—in the past, behind me. In Jesus' name, I pray, Amen.

Chapter 3

Preparing for Change

*"Put on the new self, created to be like God in
true righteousness and holiness."*

—Ephesians 4:24

My friend, Michael, is a 42-year-old man, who is 5'7" tall, and weighs 326 pounds. He has an 8-year history of Type 2 diabetes and frequently complains of fatigue, difficulty losing weight, and depression.

He has noticed a marked decrease in his energy level, particularly after lunch. He realizes that he has gained a tremendous amount of weight since being placed on insulin 7 years ago. His weight has continued to rise over the past 6 years, and he is presently at the highest weight he has ever been. He says that every time he tries to cut down on his eating he feels shaky and unstable. He does not follow any specific diet and has been so fearful of hypoglycemia that he often eats extra snacks.

His doctor has repeatedly advised him to lose weight and exercise to improve his health status. He complains that the pain in his knees and ankles makes it difficult to do any exercise. In addition to being a diabetic, Michael also suffers from sleep apnea, high blood pressure, and elevated cholesterol.

Upon his last visit to the doctor, Michael received a huge wake up call. Instead of reporting the results of his last physical, the doctor simply looked him in the eye and said, "Change or die."

Although Michael wants to change, he does not know how. He knows that the food he is eating is having a negative impact on his health, but he is stuck in a cyclical and destructive pattern that he does not know how to get out of.

Many of us are like Michael. We repeatedly eat foods that we know are not good for us. This type of eating results in negative consequences like joint pain, chronic fatigue, food allergies, lethargy, obesity, diabetes, heart disease, acid reflux, etc. This type of eating also manifests in mental, emotional, and social disorders that disrupt our lives. But, despite these challenges, we still continue to engage in negative eating patterns because we would rather suffer with certain health conditions than give up the foods that we have grown to love.

That's the bad news. Here's the good news: You can reverse, remediate, or improve most, if not all, adverse health conditions. You can adopt a healthy lifestyle that will afford you the simple pleasures you desire - like playing with your children/ grandchildren in the park, like wearing an outfit without squeezing into it, like walking up a flight of stairs without getting winded, like eating without relying on medication to stabilize your blood sugar levels, or like attending your high school/college reunion and being proud of your appearance. Yes, you have the power to create the life that you want. All you have to do is make the decision to change. And when you change what you know, you will change what you do.

Write three things that you want to change about your health:

____

____

____

Prayer:

Lord, You have said to call upon You in the day of trouble and You will deliver us. I call upon You now and ask that You would set me free from negative eating habits. If this deliverance is not immediate, keep me from discouragement and help me to remain confident that You have begun a good work in me and will complete it. When I feel that things are hopeless, help me to remember that what I cannot change in my own strength, You can-- for all things are possible with you. In Jesus' name, I pray. Amen.

Chapter 4

Making Healthier Choices

"Therefore prepare your minds for action, be self controlled; set your hope fully on the grace to be given you when Jesus Christ is revealed."

—*1 Peter 1:13*

Have you ever made a New Year's resolution? When you make a resolution you make a firm decision to make a change. In terms of your health, you may resolve to lose 50lbs, or to give up junk food, or to get more rest. I'm here to tell you that those resolutions won't work for 3 reasons:

First, resolutions are too overwhelming. Monumental tasks like these need to be broken down into smaller stages. For example, if you want to lose 50lbs. you must break that goal down into steps. Step one might be to wake up 15 minutes earlier so that you can eat breakfast at home. Step two might be to change your hours at work so that you have time to come home, make dinner, and eat before 7:00 p.m. Step three may be to take the stairs instead of the elevator, or park your car 15 feet further from where you usually park so that you will get a little more exercise.

In other words, it's not about will power, it's about gradually changing your habits to accommodate a healthier lifestyle. For example, a friend of mine, who is always attracted to the same type of man, always ends up getting hurt. When the relationship ends, she repeatedly asks, "Why does this always happen to me?" Well the truth of the matter is you can't continue to make the same choices and expect different results. The solution to her problem is not having the will power to avoid men, her solution lies in analyzing her choices, looking at the results, and then choosing differently. What is true about relationships is also true about food. You can't continue to eat a ten pack of Twinkies at twelve midnight and expect to lose 50 lbs. You have to make different choices.

The second reason why resolutions won't work is because people don't have the right information to accomplish their task. I can attest to this. I was once 48lbs. overweight. I dieted. I exercised. I wore plastic thermal sweat suits. I drank miracle diet drinks. Some of these things worked for a while, but most of them didn't. It wasn't because I was weak or a failure. It was because I did not have the right information. Hosea 4:6 says "My people perish for a lack of knowledge." To say it more simply, if you knew better, you would do better. It wasn't until I began to investigate and read books, pray for wisdom, and seek counsel that I was able to figure out what worked best for me.

The third reason why resolutions fail is because people want instant results. If you want to turn your resolution into a reality then you must put in the time. Although we have been cultivated in a microwave society, with certain things, there are no short cuts. Change requires preparation and takes time. For example, every morning I make my breakfast and lunch before leaving the house because there are very limited food choices around my place of work. I know that if I don't prepare my food at home, I will probably make an unhealthy choice. So, packing my lunch has become part of my daily routine. Just like brushing my teeth or taking a shower, I will not leave the house without my lunch in tow. Even though I have to wake up ½ hour earlier to do this, I sacrifice the time on a consistent basis to get the desired results.

Here are 3 practices that will help facilitate change in your eating lifestyle:

1. **Stock Your Cabinets/Fridge with Healthy Foods:** Have you ever heard the expression, "out of sight, out of mind?" Well, it really is true. Even retailers take advantage of this psychological construct by placing "impulse" items by the check-out counter to boost profits. With this in mind, you must make a conscious decision to control your fridge and pantry by stocking up on healthy foods and snacks. If cookies, candy, soda, and chips aren't in your kitchen then you won't be tempted to indulge. Fill up your fridge/cupboards with fresh fruits, whole grains, and vegetables. On occasion, buy snacks from the health food store, but be sure to read the labels. Just because the item is in a health food store, doesn't mean that it is actually healthy. Look for items that have fewer ingredients, a lower fat content, and less sugar than more mainstream choices. Also remember, that sugar is often disguised by other names. Any ingredient ending in the suffix "-ose" is actually sugar, (for example, high fructose corn syrup, dextrose, maltose, glucose, galactose, etc.)

2. **Carry Healthy Snacks:** If you are going to be out of the house for a long period of time, be sure to plan ahead. Pack up and carry healthy snacks at all times!

Enjoy a box of raisins, a yogurt, an apple or some carrot sticks. If you are not proactive in this way, when you become hungry you will reach for whatever is readily available: chips from the vending machine, candy on your co-workers desk, etc. While it's easy to grab these items, the added sugar, calories, and fat they contain will wreak havoc on both your heart and waistline. When consuming these types of treats, it's important to remember—a moment on the lips, a lifetime on the hips!

3. **Eat regularly:** Oftentimes, we consume too little in order to overcompensate for the times we have consumed too much. We assume that the "fast-after feasting" method is best. But, the reality is, starving ourselves today only makes us hungrier tomorrow. Although, there are times when God call us to a spiritual fast, we need to make sure that our motivations for not eating are clear.

Everyone's heard the old adage that breakfast is the most important meal of the day. Well, it's true. If you split the word "breakfast" into two parts you have the words "break" and "fast." So, essentially, when you eat breakfast, you are *breaking your fast.* If you skip breakfast, you are forcing your body to remain in "storing fat" mode. When you take that first bite in the morning, the storage stops and your metabolism gets a jolt. But, be selective with your breakfast choices. Sweet breakfast cereals, bagels, pancakes, toaster treats, and other sugar laden meals are tempting, but the initial sugar high they supply will usually cause you to "crash" a short time later. For a high-energy day, fill up on fiber and/or protein. Stay away from sugar, particularly early in the morning. Oatmeal (slow cooked, not instant), eggs, plain yogurt with fresh fruit, or a freshly juiced green drink, are much better choices that will help to stabilize your blood sugar level.

If breakfast is the most important meal of the day, then lunch runs a close second. You'll be less likely to nibble on the munchies displayed at your 2:00 meeting if you have just eaten a wholesome lunch at noon. Make sure you take time out of your busy day to eat a healthy lunch, and always attend meetings on a full stomach!

It has been said that there are two pains in life: The pain of regret and the pain of discipline. While initially it may be painful to get up earlier to make your lunch or go to the gym three times a week, these practices will give you what you desire. And I can attest to the fact, if you are not disciplined you will certainly regret it!

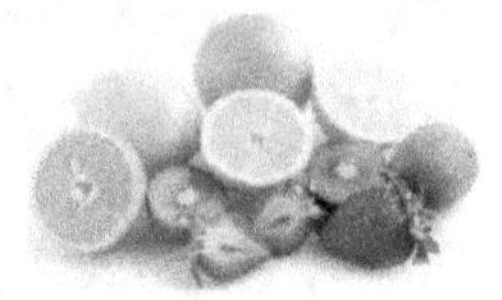

If breakfast is the most important meal of the day, then lunch runs a close second. You'll be less likely to nibble on the munchies displayed at your 2:00 meeting if you have just eaten a wholesome lunch at noon. Make sure you take time out of your busy day to eat a healthy lunch, and always attend meetings on a full stomach!

Write down three practices you are currently doing that are unhealthy.

____

____

____

Write down three things that you should be doing to improve your health.

Prayer:

Father God, grant me the wisdom to determine what goals I should set for myself when it comes to realistic weight loss. Help me to set small, attainable goals that I will be able to achieve. Give me the strength I need to admit that I can't do this in a hurry. Help me to remember that this journey has nothing to do with will power, but everything to do with planning, preparation, and prayer. Thank you for Your guidance, Your power, and Your mercy. In Jesus' mighty name I pray. Amen.

Part Three: The Body

Chapter 1

Choosing Proper Foods – Dietary Guidelines

"So obey the commands, laws and rules I'm giving you today. If you listen to these rules and faithfully obey them, the LORD your God will keep his promise to you and be merciful to you, as he swore to your ancestors."

—Deuteronomy 7:12-15, NIV

In Genesis 9:3 God declares, "Everything that lives and moves will be food for you. Just as I gave you the green plants, I now give you everything." And although God clearly established that man had dominion over the plants and animals on the earth, today we pay thousands of dollars to rehabilitate individuals who are dominated and controlled by food and plant substances!

In fact, did you ever realize that the very first sin occurred with food? Not only did Adam and Eve affect the course of history with their indulgence in the forbidden fruit, but they set a precedent of eating things that God deems off limits. Just as God cautioned Adam and Eve about eating from the "tree of knowledge," He also warns us about the consequences of eating certain foods: "You are therefore to make a distinction between the clean animal and the unclean, and between the unclean bird and the clean; and you shall not make yourselves detestable by animal or by bird or by anything that creeps on the ground, which I have separated for you as unclean" (Leviticus 20:25, NIV). However, for many Christians food has emerged as the vice of choice. Because pre-marital sex, drugs, and alcohol are "forbidden" in the Christian community, many Christians self-medicate with food. But, what some fail to realize is that food is just as addictive!

Food is a powerful drug. In fact, it may be the most powerful drug you will ever take. However, like any drug, food can help you or harm you depending on how you use it. Used correctly, food can make you more energized and healthier with the guarantee of a longer more active life. Used *incorrectly*, food can become your worst enemy –robbing you of a healthy body, healthy weight and a healthy mind. Most importantly, if food is used improperly, it can also shorten your life.

The Bible imparts simple instructions, sound principles and clear guidelines regarding the foods designed for our health and happiness: (1) Trees whose edible yield is bearing seed or is seeds (i.e.: apples, avocados, grapefruit, pecans, papaya, cherries, olives, walnuts); (2) Plants whose edible yield is bearing seed or is seeds (i.e. Tomatoes, beans, lentils, wheat, berries, squash, corn, rye); (3) Field plants – herbs, roots, leafy vegetables (ie. Greens, onions, sweet potatoes, carrots, parsley, cabbage, celery); and (4) clean meat (see the chart on the next page):

Clean Meat List		
Land Animals	**Birds of the Air & Fowl**	**Lake, River & Sea Life**
Buffalo Cow Deer Reindeer Antelope Gazelles Goats Rams Lamb Sheep Elks Moose Caribou	Chickens Turkeys Partridges Sparrows Doves Ducks Geese Pheasants Quail	Trout Tuna Salmon Halibut Bluegills Sunfish Cod Fish Flounder Perch Herring Sardines Bass Smelt Mackerel Tilapia

The Biblical dietary restrictions regarding clean meat are easy to understand. For land animals to be considered clean, they must both chew the cud and have a cloven (divide) hoof. Fish must have both scales and fins. In general, birds are considered clean. The exceptions include birds of prey, bats, winged insects (except grasshoppers), scavenger birds, etc.

Now, many of you will notice that there is no shell fish on the list. This is because shell fish are considered to be scavengers of the sea. They come in two categories: mollusks and crustaceans. Animals in the crustacean family include barnacles, crabs, crayfish, lobsters, prawns, shrimps, water fleas and wood lice. Animals in the mollusk family include chitons, clams, conch, cuttlefish, limpets, octopus, oysters, scallops, slugs, squid, and whelk.

Whether a mollusk or crustacean, all shellfish live on the sea floor where there is a large amount of bacteria and toxins. In addition, many shellfish, such as clams and oysters, are filter feeders and have a tendency to accumulate these chemical substances in their bodies.

The Food and Drug Administration (FDA) estimates that 5-10% of raw mollusks coming to market are contaminated with Vibrio, a type of bacteria which can cause food borne illnesses. In addition, paralytic shellfish poisoning (PSP) although not as common, is still a potential danger when shelled sea life, that can cause paralysis and even death to its victims, is consumed.

To be on the safe side, try substituting shellfish with other proteins.

Choosing Proper Foods –Health Tips

Agriculture is a common theme in the Bible. The fruits of God and bountiful harvests came from good soil. Food was unrefined and whole. After World War II came the advent of chemical farming and food processing. Today, most of the soils and foods throughout much of the world have been depleted of vitamins, nutrients and other minerals. Additionally, our food supply is also full of pollutants and farm chemicals. The modern denaturing of foods through refining and chemical treatment has rendered them incapable of fostering equilibrium and health. As a result, we must take precautions when making food choices.

The following is a list of criteria that should be considered before food consumption takes place.

The Majority of Food Should Be:

1. **Seasonal** – In Act 14:17, it states, "...He did good

49

and gave you rains from heaven and fruitful seasons, satisfying your hearts with food and gladness." It's important to keep the seasons in mind when choosing certain foods. Vegetables and fruits should be grown locally and in season whenever possible. Nature has a way of considering the climate and producing foods that our bodies need at the perfect time. For instance, a watermelon ripens in the summer and proves to be a refreshing treat on a hot day. Also, we benefit from stocking up on the foods that ripen in late autumn to ensure staying healthy during the winter. Although it is great to have exotic fruit occasionally, many imported vegetables and fruits are picked well before they are fully ripened. Moreover, preservatives are usually added.

2. **Whole** – Whole foods are foods that nature provides, with all of their edible parts. Whole foods of vegetable origin include fresh fruits and vegetables, whole grains (brown rice, whole wheat, buckwheat, rye, cornmeal, millet, quinoa, and oats), beans and legumes (kidney beans, chick peas, lentils), nuts and seeds. Whole foods that are of animal origin include small whole fish (like sardines), eggs, and small fowl (like a cornish hen). These are foods that you can typically consume in one setting. On the other hand, fragmented foods include all of the foods that are missing original parts. To better understand the concept of fragmented food, think about it this way: a cow is whole, a steak is fragmented. (You may notice that both the fragmented and whole foods are the same foods listed previously in the Biblical food regimen). Fragmented food is okay, but processed foods (an extreme case of

fragmentation) are to be avoided. When foods are processed, manufacturers take a large portion of whole food and condense it into a large amount of calories. For example, a large potato has roughly 200 calories. A pound of potatoes have approximately 500 calories. But, if you take a potato, dry it, ground it, shape it, and fry it, you will almost triple the calorie count! Did you know that one pound of Pringles potato chips has 2,500 calories? In addition to adding weight, processed foods make glucose levels increase, and insulin levels rise. So, whenever possible, eat foods the way they were created by nature. Often times, the best phytonutrients and vitamins are found in the rind, pod, and/or seeds. When choosing a food, ask yourself, "Did God make it this way?" Keep in mind, there is no such thing as a Twinkie tree! So, if it doesn't rot or sprout, throw it out!

3. **Organic** – Originally, all foods were organic – grown and prepared without herbicides, pesticides, chemicals, hormones, etc. Our food today, whether of vegetable or animal origin, is not only deficient in nutrients but it is also ridden with pollutants and chemicals. For this reason, it is imperative to always wash vegetables and fruits thoroughly before eating them. I recommend using a fruit and vegetable wash from your local health food store or you can make your own using the following formula: 1 cup of white vinegar, 1 cup of water, ½ juice of a lemon, 1 tablespoon of baking soda. Mix these ingredients and pour the solution into a spray bottle for convenience. This process removes harmful waxes, pesticides, and/or other impurities that may be present. Also, if

you eat dairy or meat products, it is essential to eat organic! Intensively reared dairy cows and farm animals are fed dangerous antibiotics, growth hormones, anti-parasite drugs and many other medications on a regular basis, whether they have an illness or not. These drugs are passed directly onto whoever consumes their dairy or meat. This can contribute to life threatening illnesses and other meat-related diseases. For those of you who refuse to pay the price of organic produce and other products, here is some food for thought (excuse the pun); the extra money you pay for organic food may save you hundreds, if not thousands of dollars in doctors' bills. It's better to pay now than pay later. You are most definitely worth it!

4. **Delicious** – If you think that eating healthy is another way of saying, "Goodbye, good food!" then you are wrong. I have often encountered people who say that they are reluctant to adopt a healthier lifestyle because it entails consuming unappealing food. Nothing is worse than eating a meal that is dull and unappetizing. So, don't! Your food should be delicious. If it is not, then you will feel deprived and you will be tempted to make unhealthy choices. It's all about making healthier swaps! You can create *tons* of recipes inspired by your favorite meals, but with much healthier ingredients. Here are a few examples:

- Instead of a glass of traditional Iced Tea, which is typically made from a refined powder loaded with sugar and preservatives, you can use herbal tea bags, water, and raw agave syrup (a natural sweetener extracted from the heart of the agave plant).

- Instead of an *Almond Joy* candy bar, which is made with sugar, milk chocolate, coconut, corn syrup, hydrogenated oils, artificial flavors and chemicals, you can make a similar snack using dates, unsweetened shredded coconut, whole almonds and carob.

- Instead of fried chicken, which is loaded with unhealthy fat, you can make crispy chicken in the oven by using chicken breasts, low-fat plain yogurt, Italian bread crumbs, and seasoning.

- Instead of making a traditional pizza, which is laden with grease, you can make a healthier pizza using a whole wheat pizza crust, olive oil, crushed tomatoes, goat cheese, mushrooms, onions, red peppers, marinated artichoke hearts, and olives.

When making these substitutions, you will probably notice that it takes less food to fill you up. This is because wholesome foods are typically higher in fiber. Hopefully, you will also discover that these alternatives are just as delicious as the traditional versions you've grown to love. So, be adventurous and turn your kitchen into a healthy eating laboratory!

Dr. Daniel Amen, author of the book, *Use Your Brain to Change Your Age*, sums it up best: Food should be CROND: Calorie Restricted and Optimally Nutritious and Delicious!

5. **Right for You** – Recently, the cashier at a local health food store approached me with a question. She asked me if I was a vegan (a strict vegetarian). She was surprised to learn that I am not – I eat fish, turkey, and eggs. When

asked the reason for her reaction, she said that she assumed that I was a vegetarian because I have a slender frame and I always purchase fresh juices, vegetable soups, and salads. I explained that at one point in my life I was a vegan, but that it did not work for me. I was always tired, cold, sluggish, and hungry! And much to my chagrin, I actually gained 13 pounds! It wasn't until I began to study nutrition, which I discovered that based on my blood type, I was actually better suited for a diet which included some animal protein. So what does this mean? It simply means that you have to find out what works for you. Using the proper food list outlined in the Bible as a framework, you can further determine what foods are most beneficial for you by examining your Blood Type. In fact, you can literally cross-reference the Biblical dietary guidelines with the Blood Type eating protocol to develop the perfect eating regimen for you. The following pages will show you how.

Prayer:

Heavenly Father, today I make a decision to change the rest of my life. I consciously choose to follow You and Your plan for my life. This includes my habits and patterns of eating. Have Your will in me, Lord. Keep me strong in You. I thank you for hearing and answering this prayer in Jesus' precious name, Amen.

Chapter 2

The Blood Type Diet

"For the life of the flesh is in the blood."

—Leviticus 17:11

Although Christians proclaim their identity in Christ, biochemically everyone on the face of the earth is a unique creation. James D'Adamo puts it this way:

> *"No two people have the same fingerprints, lip prints, or voice prints...Because I felt that all people were different from one another, I did not think it was logical that they should eat the same foods. It became clear to me that since each person was housed in a special body with different strengths, weaknesses, and nutritional requirements, the only way to maintain health or cure illness was to accommodate that particular patient's specific needs."*

James D'Adamo's son, Peter, a naturopathic doctor, is the author of *Eat Right for Your Type*, one of the most popular weight loss protocols to date. In this book, D'Adamo asserts that the blood type is the most critical factor in determining a healthy diet. As a result, he has developed four distinct diets for each blood type: A, B, O, and AB.

- **Blood Type O diet:** Type O's should consume a higher protein diet and limit the consumption of grains, breads, legumes, and beans.

- **Blood Type A diet:** Unlike Type O's, Type A's should avoid meat and eat high amounts of vegetables. They should also avoid dairy and wheat products.

- **Blood Type B diet:** Type B's have a strong immune system and a flexible digestive system. They are the only ones who can thrive on dairy products (except for those who are lactose intolerant). Foods to be avoided are lentils and wheat.

- **Blood Type AB diet:** Type AB's are a mixture of blood types A and B, meaning they are primarily vegetarian but have a reasonable amount of grains, protein and dairy as part of daily dietary intake.

The underlying principle of this dietary protocol is that different blood types digest food proteins or lectins differently. If you eat foods containing lectins that are incompatible with your blood type, you may experience a slower metabolism, bloating, inflammation, or even diseases such as lupus or cancer. According to the developer of this diet the best way to avoid these effects is to eat foods that are specifically prescribed for your blood type.

When following this food plan, the first thing you have to do is determine your blood type, if you do not already know it. This can be done a few ways: (1) you could donate blood to the

Red Cross and request a donor card, (2) you can ask your doctor to test for your blood type, or (3) you can purchase a "blood typing kit", over the Internet, and test yourself.

When beginning this dietary plan, you should start slowly. Proceed in small increments in order to guarantee success. Gradually integrate the plan into your daily life so that it becomes habitual. Also, you do not have to give up every "forbidden" food as soon as you begin. Rather, I suggest that you slowly wean yourself off a few foods every week and find creative substitutes.

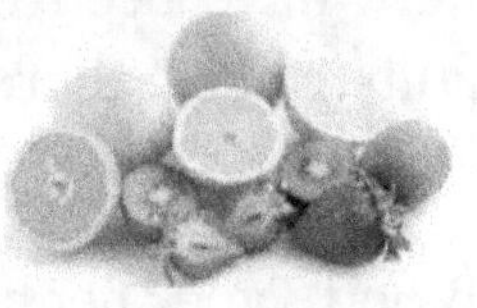

The best way to avoid adverse effects to your body and health is to eat foods that are specifically prescribed for your blood type. If you choose to eat according to your blood type, please remember that you may need to make adjustments that best suit your unique nutritional needs. Consult your doctor and a nutritionist.

Because many of you have children and spouses you have to consider, try to adhere to the plan as much as you can without putting stress on your household relations or creating a sense of inconvenience. Practice substituting wholesome foods that you enjoy for the 'avoid' foods as much as possible. Plan your meals in advance so that the transition goes smoothly for you. Nothing is worse than getting ready to prepare a meal and realizing that some of the ingredients fall into the banned category!

Although this plan may seem too restrictive, I have found it to be very effective. Before learning about this protocol, I was under the impression that if I was a vegan I would lose weight.

But, I quickly learned that that was a flagrant misconception. This plan really helped me to understand why I felt so weak and unstable as a vegan and why my health improved tremendously when I added animal food to my diet. It was also the first eating regimen that helped me to effectively lose weight and keep it off. I have used this plan with all of my clients and have found it to be 90% accurate (occasionally, there have been instances in which certain medical conditions like thyroid issues, medications, and illnesses have skewed results).

The official website for the Blood Type Diet has a myriad of resources that will help you in this process, as well as a helpful member community that can answer any questions you may have while on the diet, if you choose to pursue it. If you are not ready to try it, definitely follow the Biblical dietary guidelines and my health tips. If you eat 70-80% of the whole foods listed in Chapter 2, you will definitely lose some weight and increase your immunity. The added benefit of cross-referencing the two eating plans is that,

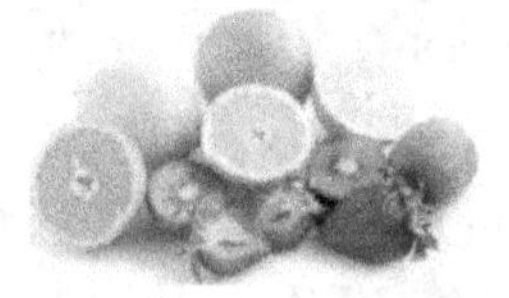

Following the Blood Type Diet combined with Biblical dietary guidelines, you are likely to lose some weight and increase your immunity. The added benefit of cross-referencing the two eating plans is that, in doing so, you would yield optimal health benefits.

in doing so, you would yield optimal health benefits. For example, when I followed the Biblical based diet, I lost 17 pounds before hitting a plateau and I experienced increased energy overall. However, when I combined the Bible diet with the Blood Type diet, I lost an additional 31 pounds, stopped experiencing inflammation in my knee and feet, regulated by blood pressure (it used to be chronically low), and recognized an improvement in my skin, hair, and nails.

Invariably, I have found that the program works. I have not yet found an energetic "O" type who is comfortable on a vegetarian diet, or an "A" type who thrived on steak! However, these recommendations are merely guidelines, not rules. If you choose to eat according to your blood type, please remember that you may need to make adjustments that best suit your unique nutritional needs.

The blood type eating protocols can be a bit overwhelming. To avoid confusion, I have included a summary sheet for each of the blood types.

TYPE AB

Strength	Weakness	Health Risk	Diet Profile	Weight Loss	Supplements
Rugged Immune System	Sensitive Digestive Tract	Heart Disease Cancer Anemia	Mixed Diet in Moderation	**Reduce:** Red meat Kidney Beans Lima Beans Seeds Corn Buckwheat	Vitamin C Hawthorn Echinacea Valerian Quercitin Milk Thistle
Combined benefits of type A and B	Allows for microbial invasion		Meat Seafood Dairy Tofu Beans Legumes Grains Vegetables Fruit	**Increase:** Tofu Fish Dairy Greens Kelp Pineapple	

Adapted from <u>Eat Right For Your Type</u> (pg. 336), New York: G.P. Putnam's Sons

TYPE A

Strength	Weakness	Health Risk	Diet Profile	Weight Loss	Supplements
Tolerant Immune System	Sensitive Digestive Tract Easily retain fluids	Heart Disease Cancer Diabetes	Vegetarian	**Reduce:** Meat Dairy Kidney Beans Lima Beans Wheat - in overabund-ance	Vitamin B Vitamin C Vitamin E Calcium
Adapts well to settled dietary and environmental conditions			Seafood Vegetables Soy	**Increase:** Vegetable Oils Soy Foods Vegetables Pineapple	

Adapted from <u>Eat Right For Your Type</u> (pg. 334), New York: G.P. Putnam's Sons

TYPE B

Strength	Weakness	Health Risk	Diet Profile	Weight Loss	Supplements
Strong Immune System Strong Nervous System	No Natural Weaknesses Tendency toward auto-immune breakdowns and rare viruses	Type 1 Diabetes Chronic Fatigue Syndrome Lou Gehrig's Disease Lupus Multiple Sclerosis	Omnivore Meat (no chicken) Dairy (unless lactose intolerant) Grains Beans Legumes Vegetables Fruit	**Reduce:** Corn Lentils Peanuts Sesame Buckwheat Wheat **Increase:** Greens Eggs Venison Liver Licorice Tea	Magnesium Licorice Gingko Lecithin

Adapted from <u>Eat Right For Your Type</u> (pg. 335), New York: G.P. Putnam's Sons

TYPE O

Strength	Weakness	Health Risk	Diet Profile	Weight Loss	Supplements
Hardy Digestive Tract Strong Immune System Efficient Metabolism	Low tolerance to new diets and new environments	Low Thyroid Function Arthritis Blood Clotting Disorders Ulcers	Red Meat Strong Enzymes to Digest Meat High Protein Vegetables Fruit	**Reduce:** Wheat/Corn/ Baked Goods Kidney Beans Navy Beans Lentils Brussels Sprouts Cauliflower Mustard	Vitamin B Vitamin K Calcium Iodine Licorice Kelp
Shorter Small Intestines Less chance for Cancer	Allows for microbial invasion		Meat Seafood Dairy Tofu Beans Legumes Grains Vegetables Fruit	**Increase:** Kelp, salt, seafood, liver, red meat, kale, spinach, broccoli	

Adapted from <u>Eat Right For Your Type</u> (pg. 333), New York: G.P. Putnam's Sons

Chapter 3

The Link Between the Bible and Blood Type

*"Now the Lord is the Spirit, and where the Spirit
of the Lord is, there is freedom."*

—2 Corinthians 3:17

As previously explored in Chapter 1, the Bible has a lot to say about nutrition and health. But, do biblical dietary laws still apply today? In the Old Testament, God outlined specific dietary laws and lists of clean and unclean foods for the Jewish people. However, the New Testament proclaims freedom from the dietary laws of the Old Testament:

*"He (Peter) became hungry and wanted
something to eat, and while the meal was being
prepared, he fell into a trance. He saw heaven
opened and something like a large sheet being
let down to earth by its four corners. It
contained all kinds of four-footed animals, as
well as reptiles of the earth and birds of the air.
Then a voice told him, "Get up, Peter. Kill and*

> *eat." (Peter replied), "Surely not, Lord...I have*
> *never eaten anything impure or unclean." The*
> *voice spoke to him a second time, "Do not call*
> *anything impure that God has made clean."*
>
> *—Acts 10:10-13*

During this period described in Acts 10, the Christian church consisted primarily of converted Jews. Although they followed the Jewish statutes, they had also accepted Jesus as the Messiah. Jewish law forbad them from having any contact with gentiles. However, God's plan was that salvation through Jesus extended to all people: Jews and gentiles. So to establish this point, God gave Peter a vision. Almost immediately afterward, a gentile, named Cornelius sent for Peter. Realizing that the vision meant that no man should be considered "impure or unclean," Peter told Cornelius about Jesus, and Cornelius became the very first gentile Christian.

Although the primary message of this story is the acceptance of gentiles into the Christian church, there is a sub level application to the Blood Type Diet. Dr. James D'Adamo has written that most of the Jewish people were Type B. The Old Testament Dietary restrictions were extremely close to the Type B food regimen. So, if the Jews followed the law, they lived healthy lives.

However, at this moment in time, Christianity was about to become a worldwide religion. What if the early Christians instructed their new gentile converts, who were Type O and Type A, which they had to subscribe to the Jewish dietary laws? The teaching that was proclaiming grace and freedom from the law, would have actually made them mentally and physically unhealthy; symbolically, they would experience mental and emotional bondage, and literally, they would be following an improper diet.

In Acts 10 and 11, God frees all blood types from the Old Testament restrictions. Although scientists would not discover Blood Types for many centuries, God knew how he created us. He protected Type As, ABs, and Os from "legalistically" trying to follow a Type B diet.

One final comment – the primary food restrictions for Jews is pork. It is also forbidden in Muslim law. Further, it is a food that appears on the "avoid" list for all of the blood types. So, I am urging all of you bacon and ham lovers to find other alternatives!

Prayer:

Father God, thank you that I am uniquely and wonderfully made. Thank you for the warm blood pumping through my veins and, thank you that this blood provides a blueprint for my individual dietary needs. Thank you for helping me to recognize that I must pay attention to how my body reacts to various foods and that there is no one-size-fits-all approach to optimal health and wellness. Thank you for your precision to detail and for knowing everything about me from the top of my head to the soles of my feet. Thank you for helping me to adopt the proper eating plan that will revitalize my body and prolong my life. In Jesus' name I pray. Amen.

Chapter 4

Keeping the Body Well-Tuned

*"A wise man is full of strength, and a man of
knowledge enhances his might."*

—*Proverbs 24:5*

One Saturday morning, after an intense workout at the gym, I stepped into a local bank. As I stood on line, I began to feel extremely warm and I broke out into a violent sweat. As the room began to spin, I spotted a vacant chair in the corner of the waiting area. With an unsteady gait, I moved toward the chair but I never reached it. I hit the floor with a loud thump and was unconscious for several seconds. When I came to, I was helped to a chair and remained there until I was well enough to walk independently.

That was the first of a series of fainting spells. Dismissing these episodes as minor occurrences, I refused to heed the advice of family and friends who urged me to seek medical attention. It wasn't until I attempted to become a blood donor that I learned that I was severely anemic. In fact, my hemoglobin count was so low that I required a blood transfusion! That was a valuable lesson for me to learn. Since then, I make it a point to undergo a yearly physical which includes a thorough blood screening. Although I encourage individuals to become their own health advocates and not rely solely on their doctor's recommendations when it comes to making decisions about their health, I do see the benefit of undergoing regular physicals.

When it comes to fine-tuning your health, put yourself in the driver's seat and take charge of your health journey. There are easy to follow health tips that will aid in taking control of your well-being:

- Have routine physicals
- Drink water
- Sleep
- Exercise

Have Routine Physicals

Next time you visit your health care provider, be sure to ask for your critical health numbers to be screened. By drawing blood, your health care provider can conduct a blood lipid profile to check your blood cholesterol, and glucose tests to check your blood sugar. Your blood pressure and weight are even easier to check with a blood pressure monitor and scales, respectively. Also, ladies, remember to ask your gynecologist to check your hormone levels. They are a great indicator of fluctuations that may drastically impact your weight, mood, body temperature, and sleep cycles.

Between doctor visits, you can monitor and track your blood sugar, blood pressure, and body weight. Easy-to-use home glucose monitors, blood pressure monitors, and bathroom scales are readily available at large discount stores and pharmacies. By keeping track of your numbers on your own, you will be able to better manage your health.

Prayer Focus:

Lord, I pray that you will help me to overcome the fear of facing my doctor with my health issues. Help me to overcome the fear of stepping on the scale and monitoring my critical numbers. Give me the courage to ask my doctor for help and advice, and instill in me the desire to advocate for my own health. Thank you for hearing and answering this prayer. In Jesus' name, I pray. Amen.

Drink Water

"And God split open the hollow place that is at Lehi, and water came out from it. And when he drank, his spirit returned, and he revived."

—Judges 15:19

My father used to always say, "Water rusts pipes." He used to drink diet drinks and juices instead of drinking water because he believed that they were healthier and more satisfying. But, truth be told, diet beverages, especially those loaded with caffeine, can increase your appetite and leave you feeling thirstier than ever! Although diet drinks are popular, they offer no nutritional benefit and they often contain harmful ingredients like aspartame, a well-known carcinogenic.

In 2009, my father was diagnosed with cancer. While I'm not suggesting that my dad contracted cancer because he didn't drink water, I do wonder why his doctors never recommended that he drink large amounts of water to help improve his condition. Even after he received his diagnosis, I never saw him drink more than a Dixie cup full of water— just enough to wash down his medication. I mention this to illustrate that many people, including my father and his medical team, underestimate the healing properties of water.

Three months after my father died, I was asked to conduct a lecture at the local library—the topic—*The Importance of Water*. I wonder if my dad would have been swayed by my presentation. Here it is in a nutshell:

The Top 10 Reasons to Drink Water:

1. Drinking pure water (free of chemicals, bacteria, and viruses) is absolutely essential to the human body's survival. A person can live for about a month without food, but only about a week without water.

2. Water helps to maintain healthy body weight by increasing metabolism and regulating appetite.

3. Water leads to increased energy levels.

4. Drinking adequate amounts of water can decrease the risk of certain types of cancer.

5. Drinking water can significantly reduce joint and/or back pain.

6. Water flushes out wastes and bacteria that cause disease.

7. Water can prevent and alleviate headaches.

8. Water naturally moisturizes skin.

9. Water aids in the digestion process and prevents constipation.

10. Water is essential for proper circulation.

As a nutritionist and radical health advocate, I implore you to give water a chance. And, if you currently drink an adequate amount of water, drink more. In fact, here is a formula you can use to help determine how much water you should be drinking on a daily basis: Your body weight divided by 2 = the amount of ounces you should consume each day. So, for example, if you weigh 160 pounds, you should drink 80 ounces of water per day. If one glass is equivalent to 8 ounces, this means that you should drink 10 glasses of water daily. I know that this may seem overwhelming if you currently don't drink much water, but you can gradually increase your water intake over time, until you reach this benchmark. In other words, start small, but by all means, START!

Prayer Focus:

Father, God, thank you for the gift of water. Help me to recognize that water has both physical and spiritual properties. Create in me the desire to use water in the physical sense to quench my thirst, nourish my cells, and revitalize my body. And help me to remember that You alone are living water, and if I trust in You I shall never thirst. I pray this prayer, in Jesus' name. Amen.

Sleep

> *"It is vain for you to rise up early, to sit up*
> *late...for so He gives His beloved sleep."*
>
> —*Psalm 127:2*

My insomnia began my freshman year of college. Each night, I would spend countless hours flirting with the notion of falling sleep. I tried everything from jumping jacks to warm milk in my attempt to shut down the committee that held my thoughts hostage every night. But, no matter what I tried, I would always end up lying face up counting each twinkling star and constellation formation projected onto my ceiling by my roommate's glow in the dark star- gazer globe.

In the bed across from me, my roommate would sleep soundly, with the exception of an occasional snore, on nights when her nose was stuffy. She, unlike me, was in complete control—she decided when she was going to sleep. I envied this control. And, even though I knew it wasn't rational, I harbored deep resentment towards her peaceful slumber. One night in a moment of sheer frustration, I became so angry by the fact that she was able to sleep, I threw a sneaker at her. And would you believe that despite this *seemingly* jarring disruption, her sleep still remained undisturbed!

Over time, I realized that I did have control. I could control the foods I consumed; I could control the time I would eat my last meal of the day; I could control what time I would go to bed; I could control the amount of light that would enter my room; I could control the temperature of the room, etc. When I made the connection, that insomnia is caused by many different factors, I began to pay attention to my daily habits. I discovered that I couldn't consume caffeinated beverages like coffee or soda hours before going to bed. I also discovered that I couldn't sleep if there was too much light in the room. When I changed my behavior, I changed my sleeping pattern. And, when I began to sleep, I experienced the following: increased immune system function, increased performance, increased level of concentration, and increased weight loss. So, if you are not sleeping, you are in effect starving your body of a basic right—the right to function effectively.

In fact, sleep is essential for good health. Although scientists don't know exactly why we need it, they know what happens when we don't get enough. Sleep deprivation leads to disease, weight gain, and premature aging. What God accomplishes within our bodies while we sleep is nothing short of miraculous. While we rest, He rebuilds and restores our cells, He replenishes our energy and reorganizes information in our brains.

The reasons for not getting enough sleep are many, and some are difficult to solve, but the Word indicates that overwork should not be one of them! (Ps 127:2) Sleep is a gift from God that we should receive with gratitude. If we're not getting enough, we need to find out why. Are we waking up too early and staying up too late to earn money to acquire things we don't need? Are we involved in activities that we think no else is capable of doing?

I'm sometimes deceived into believing that the work I do when I'm awake is far more important than the work God does while I'm asleep. Essentially, refusing God's gift of sleep is like telling Him that our work is more important than His. Remember, God does not want anyone to become a slave to work. He wants us to enjoy His gift of sleep. Minister Vance Havner sums it up best, "If we do not come apart and rest awhile, we may just come apart."

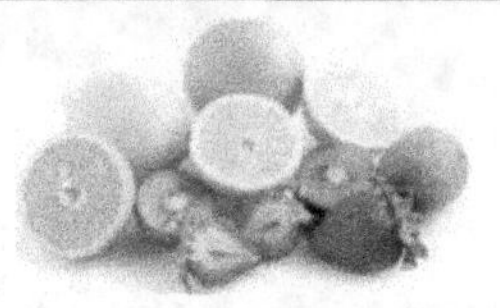

Insomnia is controllable. You could control the foods you consume, the time you eat your last meal of the day, the time you would go to bed, the amount of light that enters your room and the temperature of the room. Insomnia is caused by many different factors. It is best to pay attention to your daily habits and learn to control those habits so your mind and body can receive the proper rest that it needs.

Prayer Focus:

Lord, grant me the wisdom to listen to wise counsel and accept sound advice. Help me to have a teachable spirit so that I am no longer a slave to old ways of thinking. Instruct me even as I am sleeping (Psalm 16:7), and in the morning, I pray that I will do what's right rather than follow the leading of my flesh. Thank you for helping to me to hear the truth and increase in knowledge. In Jesus' name I pray. Amen.

Exercise

> *"Or do you not know that your body is a temple of the Holy Spirit within you, whom you have from God? You are not your own, for you were bought with a price. So glorify God in your body."*
>
> —*1 Corinthians 6:19-20*

Growing up, I never liked to exercise. In high school, my lowest grade was always in Physical Education. Twice a week, I would come up with any and every excuse not to participate in gym class. Typically, I would have cramps, be unprepared, or would feign an injury. Sometimes the teacher would buy it, but most of the time she would not.

Why did I go to such great lengths to avoid participating in gym class, you may ask? Because gym class highlighted my biggest deficiency--athleticism! While I excelled academically, when it came to physical activity, I failed miserably! In fact, the only reason why I passed phys ed class at all was because I would always score 95% or better on the written exams. Yes, although I knew all of the rules of engagement, I could not physically execute them!

I began to exercise consistently and continuously when I made the connection that exercise would make a dramatic difference in my personal life. For thirty years, I suffered from debilitating menstrual cramps. Every 28 days, I would have to take a day off from work or school because I was unable to stand up straight. One day my doctor told me that if I exercised vigorously for a minimum of 30 minutes a day, it would make a big difference in my monthly cycle. I followed his advice and was pleasantly surprised by the results. Ever since I started exercising regularly, the pain has diminished significantly. I also have increased energy and a leaner physique to boot!

Even though everyone knows that exercise is beneficial, a lot of us don't do it for various reasons. While my excuse was grounded in insecurity, other excuses may be related to time, pain, or money. Whatever the condition, excuse, or issue, I'm here to tell you that you CAN exercise in one way or another. All exercise can be modified to fit your unique situation. Start, even if you just tap your toes. Do what you can and increase gradually. I promise you things will improve right away.

For those of you who do not currently exercise, please heed the following advice before beginning an exercise regimen:

First, tell your health care professional what you plan to do. Talk about any restrictions or modifications that may be advisable.

Next, get a comfortable pair of sneakers to protect your feet. Find comfortable clothes, not too tight and not too loose. Cotton works best.

Finally, I encourage you to take a class. Classes are easy to find and are generally offered at local gyms and recreation centers, YMCA's, YWCA's, or wellness centers. Look for classes labeled: beginner, easy, gentle, basic, low impact, etc. Once you find a class you think you might like--try it. You may be able to participate for free. If not, you may be able to pay for just one class.

Speak to the instructor before class, and tell him/her whatever physical challenges you may have. He/she will guide you and help prevent you from sustaining any injuries. During the class, you will probably meet like-minded people who can help support you on this new journey.

If you do not want to take a class, then turn what you love into exercise. Dance, swim, play tennis, walk, jog, or garden. It doesn't matter what you do, just do something!

Three cautions:

Never do anything that hurts! If you experience discomfort shortly after exercise or even the next day, ice it, and the tension should lessen. If the discomfort lasts two days, then you worked too hard. Don't exert as much energy during your next session.

Starting to exercise now is a big step. I know. I've done it. Others have done it. You can do it too. Exercise is now considered to be the most important lifestyle component for managing your health. Quality food, adequate amounts of water, ample sleep, are all important—but exercise is critical for the quality of your life, for the rest of your life.

To drive my point home, I make this analogy: What do the Super Bowl and exercise have in common? During the Super Bowl there are 22,000,000 people who **need** exercise watching 22 who don't! The time has come for you to stop sitting on the sidelines--take action now!

Prayer Focus:

Lord, I thank you for the desire you have placed in my heart to become physically fit. Grant me the wisdom to adopt the most appropriate form of exercise, one that fits my lifestyle and needs, and one that I will enjoy. Help me to continue what I start even when it becomes challenging, and take away the excuses when I am tempted to return to my old ways. I pray this prayer in Jesus' name, Amen.

Conclusion

"Choose my instruction instead of silver,
knowledge rather than choice gold, for wisdom
is more precious than rubies, and nothing you
desire can compare with her."

—Proverbs 8: 10-11

Recently, I saw a commercial for a popular restaurant chain that made an amazing claim: "Help Yourself to Happiness." Wouldn't it be something if a serving of pasta, chicken or sweet potato pie would be all that was needed to provide happiness? Even though no eatery can fulfill this promise, often times our pursuit of happiness *does* involve food. How many times have you reached for the chocolate chip cookies to pacify yourself after enduring an emotional hurt? How many times have you turned to the Doritos when you were feeling blue? But, the reality is when food is used to garner brief moments of pleasure, satisfaction, or distraction, the cry of our hearts remains unheard—the cry for help and hope. Psalm 146:5 says it best, "Happy is he who has the God of Jacob for his help, whose hope is in the Lord his God."

We must always remember that our challenges aren't against flesh and blood; neither are the solutions to these challenges. We can't combat spiritual forces with ice cream or pie, just like we can't try to solve our problems by eating them away. In order to resolve our issues, we have to reach out to "Someone" instead of "something." In times of despair we must learn to overlook the Oreos and reach out for Jesus instead. For it is only when we trust in God that we can find the happiness we so desperately desire.

And so, yes, help yourself. Help yourself to a double portion of health, healing, and wholeness by developing a close, personal relationship with Christ. Ask Him to help you to use food the way He designed it to be used. Ask him to help you to submit your problems to Him and to look to Him for the solutions. For, He is the only source of true wisdom and intelligence. And, thankfully, He has deposited His Spirit in you. As you make the decision to adopt a healthier lifestyle, embrace the fact that God loves you, and when you ask Him for help, He will teach you all things (1 John 2:27).

Prayer

God, thank you for placing in me the desire to take care of my body, to eat the kind of food that brings health, to get regular exercise, and avoid anything that would be harmful to me. Help me to understand that my body is a temple and that I should care for it as such. Please remind me that this is a joyful journey and not a never-ending diet. Help me to enjoy this new lifestyle change that will bring me health and wholeness. Thank you, in Jesus' name, Amen.

Bibliography

Amen, Daniel, M.D., *Use Your Brain to Change Your Age*, Little, Brown Book Group, London, 2012.

D'Adamo, Peter J., M.D., *Eat Right For Your Type*, G.P. Putnam's Sons, New York, N.Y., 1997.

Frahm, Dave, *Healthy Habits*, Pinon Press, Colorado Springs, CO, 1993.

Gittleman, Ann Louise, *Your Body Knows Best*, Pocket Books, New York, NY 1997.

Russel, Rex, M.D., *What the Bible Says About Healthy Living*, Regal Books, Ventura, CA, 1996.

Tessler, Gordon S., Ph.D., *The Genesis Diet*, Be Well Publications, Raleigh, NC, 1996

White, Paula, Deal With It!: *You Cannot Conquer What You Will Not Confront*, Thomas Nelson, Nashville, TN, 2005.

http://www.josephprince.com/365-break-every-bad-habit-with-Christ.

http://www.fda.gov/downloads/Food/GuidanceRegulation/U
CM252448.pdf

Keri's Journey

After being prodded and poked by countless doctors and health care professionals, and spending thousands of dollars on prescriptions, remedies, and concoctions, Keri Watkins Webb was sick and tired of being sick and tired. As she began to seek spiritual counsel for her health issues she was directed to the Bible verse, "Beloved, above all, I wish that ye prosper and be in good health even as your soul prospers."(3 John 2). After meditating on this scripture, Keri came to the realization that her body was the vehicle through which she could physically manifest God's will—and in order to do His will, her body had to be strong. With this new insight, she began her spiritual and physical journey toward holistic health and healing. After modifying her eating habits, increasing her exercise regimen and relying on spiritual guidance, she overcame numerous health conditions that plagued her body and impacted her life: hypothyroidism, radon poisoning, and a persistent weight problem—just to name a few.

In May 2005, she was led to share her knowledge and experience with others. She opened a fitness center for women and developed a holistic health ministry grounded in the belief that health is the vehicle that allows you to fulfill God's purpose for your life. She believes that once you experience good health, you will feel truly blessed, and will bless others in return.

About Keri

Keri Watkins Webb is a nutritionist, educator, lecturer, author and lifestyle coach committed to transforming the fatally flawed, American health care system by providing safe and practical solutions to people's health problems. Over the past 15 years, she has encouraged healthy, mindful living and has inspired individuals to take control of their health rather than relying solely on the recommendations of medical doctors. Keri believes that everyone can become their own health expert once they make the connection that their mind, body and spirit are intricately linked. By partnering with her clients, she teaches them how to tap into their own instincts and abilities so that they can function independently and confidently. She believes that once people are empowered to strengthen themselves, they will, in turn, strengthen their communities.

Keri has found great success in promoting time-tested holistic approaches and by *teaching* her clients what to do, instead of *telling* them what to do. After participating in Keri's whole-body approach to wellness, her clients have experienced improved immunity, increased energy, significant weight loss and optimal health.

Keri is a certified Holistic Health Coach with training in Eastern and Western nutritional theory from the Institute of Integrative Nutrition in NYC. She also holds a Master's Degree in Holistic Health Studies from Georgian Court

University and a Certificate in Christian Ministry from New York Theological Seminary. In 2010, she founded Empowered Living, LLC, a holistic healthcare practice dedicated to educating, invigorating, and rejuvenating the mind, body, and spirit. Currently, she teaches Nutrition at Empire State College and counsels a sizable number of clients from her offices in Brooklyn and Queens, New York.

www.ingramcontent.com/pod-product-compliance
Lightning Source LLC
Chambersburg PA
CBHW070816240726
48654CB00007B/377